MW00896004

Contents

1 Useful Terms

2 Frankincense

4 Lavender

6 Peppermint

8 Lemon

10 Copaiba

12 Myrrh

14 Wintergreen

16 Spearmint

18 Cedarwood

20 Ginger

22 Lemongrass

24 Patchouli

26 Oregano

28 Orange

30 Cinnamon

32 Helichrysum

34 Nutmeg

36 Sandalwood

38 Ylang Ylang

40 Marjoram

42 Rosemary

44 Black Spruce

46 Grapefruit

48 Vetiver

50 Clove

52 Bergamot

54 Melaleuca

56 Lime

58 Eucalyptus

60 Chamomile

62 Summary

Dear Guidebook User,

I am very happy that you have a copy of this guidebook as it will help you on your journey to learning about the amazing benefits of essential oils! Handle this guidebook with extreme care. Many of the incredible secrets of the Essential Heroes are contained within these pages and you must make sure that they do not fall into the wrong hands. It is recommended that you review the material within these pages often so you will be able to assist the Essential Heroes when they need your help fighting the many dangers and toxins present in the world! Remember, essential oils are powerful and should never be used without the help of an adult! Happy reading!!!

-Fredrick Frankincense

Useful Terms

Essential Oil: The most important and powerful parts of a plant in liquid form.

Steam Distilled: A process where pieces of a plant are steamed (like when you cook vegetables) to help the essential oils come out of the plant material so we can use them.

Cold Pressed: Instead of being steamed, citrus essential oils are squeezed from plant material by heavy presses.

Support: One of the main ways essential oils work is by supporting our bodies to do what they were designed to do.

Fredrick Frankincense

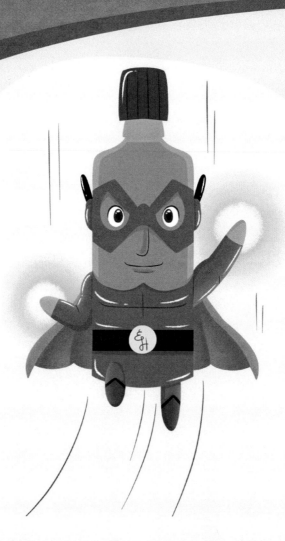

Common Uses for Frankincense:
- Calming
- Skin Soothing
- Immune Support

Where in the world?

Frankincense oil comes from thick resin collected from Frankincense trees mostly found in the Middle East.

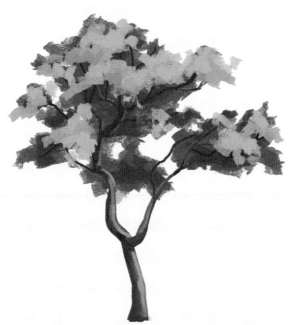

Smell
Rich
Deep

Essential Facts
People in ancient cultures used to chew frankincense resin like bubble gum!!!

Lucy Lavender

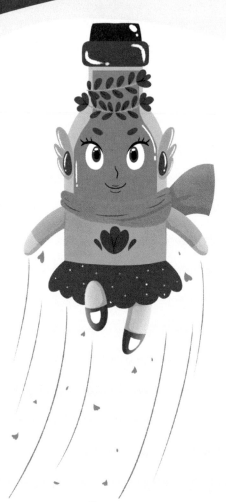

Common Uses for Lavender:
- Skin Soothing
- Emotional Support
- Calming

Where in the world?

Lavender oil is distilled from the entire plant found in Europe, North Africa, the Mediterranean, and North America.

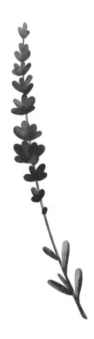

Essential Facts

Honeybees love lavender blossoms, and hives near lavender fields produce excellent, sweet honey!!!

Smell

Floral
Sweet

Penelope Peppermint

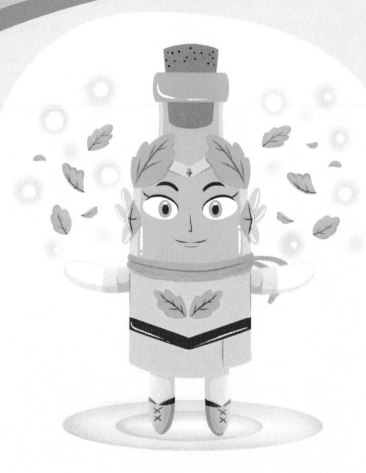

Common Uses for Peppermint:
- Cooling
- Tummy Soothing
- Stimulating

Where in the world?

Peppermint oil is distilled from peppermint leaves found mainly in the Middle East and Europe.

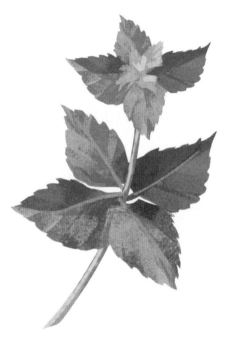

Smell

Minty
Intense

Essential Facts

Peppermint is the number one seller of all candy flavors (other than chocolate) in the world!!!

Lisa Lemon

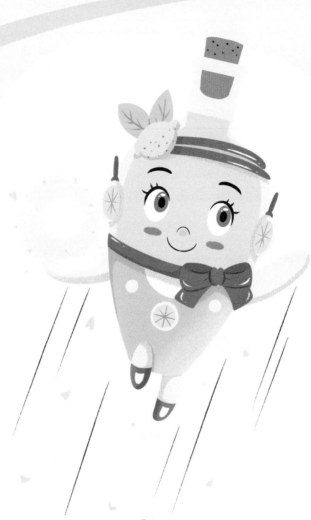

Common Uses for Lemon:
- Uplifting
- Emotional Support
- Cleansing

Where in the world?

Lemon oil comes from the rind of the lemon and is most commonly found in Asia, Italy, and parts of North America.

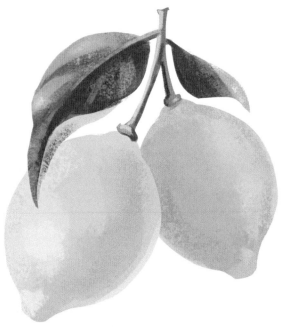

Essential Facts
It takes about 75 lemons to make a single bottle of lemon essential oil!!!

Smell
Sweet
Citrusy

Coby Copaiba

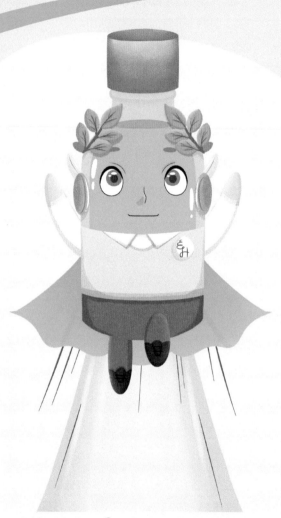

Common Uses for Copaiba:
- Calming
- Joint Support
- Muscle Soothing

Where in the world?

Copaiba oil comes from the resin
of the copaiba tree found in the Amazon
regions of Brazil and Ecuador.

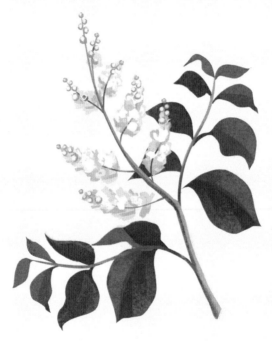

Smell

Soft
Sweet

Essential Facts

Copaiba resin is harvested
the same way as maple
syrup: tapping into the
tree and waiting for
buckets to fill!!!

Marvin Myrrh

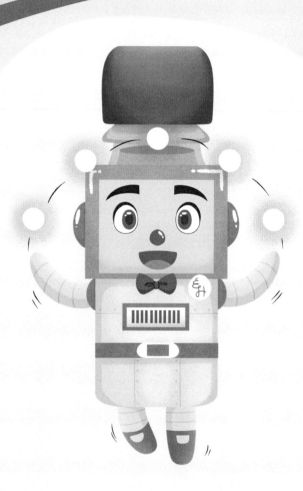

Common Uses for Lemon:
- Skin Health
- Calming
- Soothing

Where in the world?

Myrrh oil is distilled from the resin of small trees found in the Middle East and Somalia.

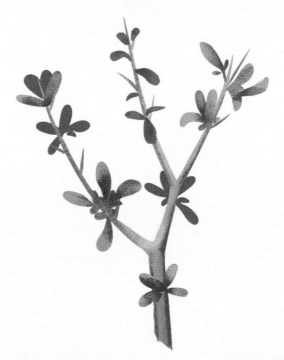

Essential Facts

Myrrh was one of the 3 gifts presented to Jesus by the wise men!!!

Smell

Warm
Earthy
Woody

Wendy Wintergreen

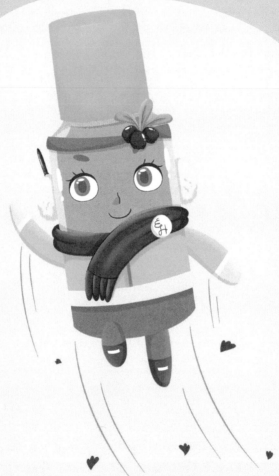

Common Uses for Wintergreen:
- Soothing
- Stimulating
- Cooling

Where in the world?

Wintergreen oil is distilled from the leaves of plants found in North America.

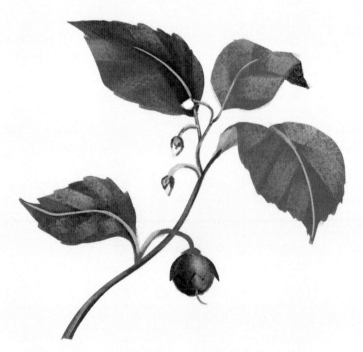

Smell
Minty
Sharp
Sweet

Essential Facts
Native Americans discovered wintergreen oil and used it for centuries for its many health supporting properties!!!

Spencer Spearmint

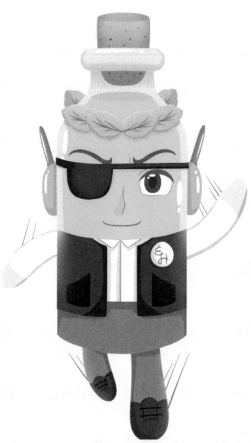

Common Uses for Spearmint:
- Energizing
- Tummy support
- Cooling

Where in the world?

Spearmint oil is distilled from the leaves of plants found in Europe, Asia, and North America.

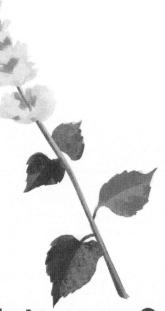

Essential Facts

Spearmint can act like a weed in vegetable gardens and flowerbeds if it can get established!!!

Smell

Minty
Sharp
Sweet

Cecelia Cedarwood

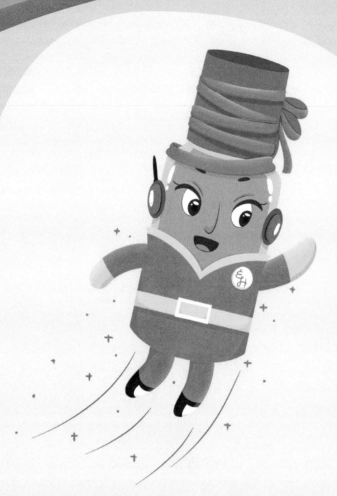

Common Uses for Cedarwood:
- Focus support
- Skin & Hair Health
- Calming

Where in the world?

Cedarwood oil is distilled from tree products found in the Mediterranean.

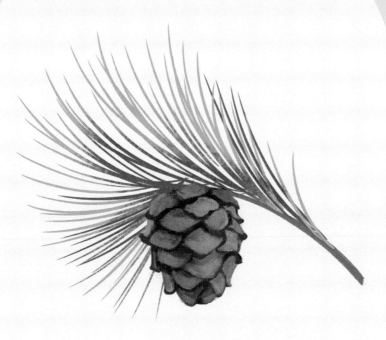

Smell
Warm
Earthy
Woody

Essential Facts
Ancient Egyptians used cedarwood oil in the mummification process because the sweet smell masked the bad odors!!!

19

Gina Ginger

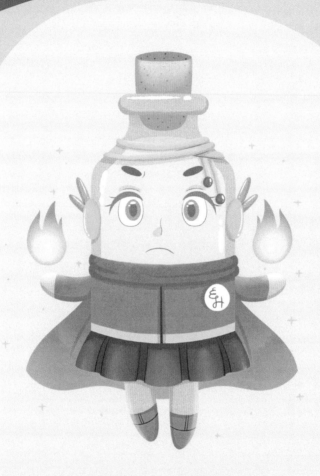

Common Uses for Ginger:
- Tummy health
- Calming
- Metabolism support

Where in the world?
Ginger oil is distilled from the roots of ginger plants found in Asia.

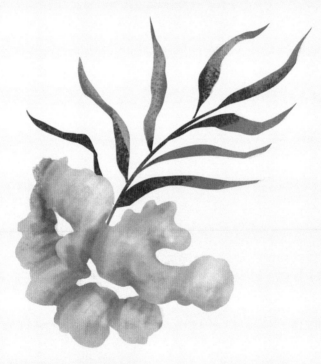

Essential Facts
Ginger has been used in India and China as a flavorful spice and digestive aid for thousands of years!!!

Smell
Spicy
Sweet
Fresh

Leon Lemongrass

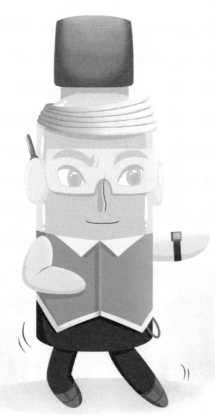

Common Uses for Lemongrass:
- Cleansing
- Soothing
- Clarity

Where in the world?
Lemongrass oil is distilled from the leaves and flowers of plants found in Asia, North Africa, and Australia.

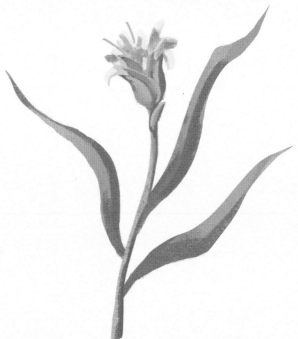

Smell
Grassy
Earthy
Bitter

Essential Facts
Lemongrass flowers are pollinated by the wind... no bees or other bugs are required!!!

Pattu Patchouli

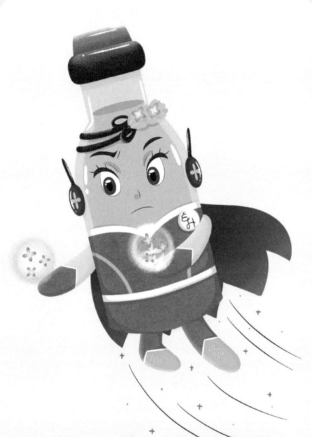

Common Uses for Patchouli:
- Skin Soothing
- Calming
- Outdoor Experience Aid

Where in the world?

Patchouli oil is distilled from the leaves and flowers of plants found in Asia.

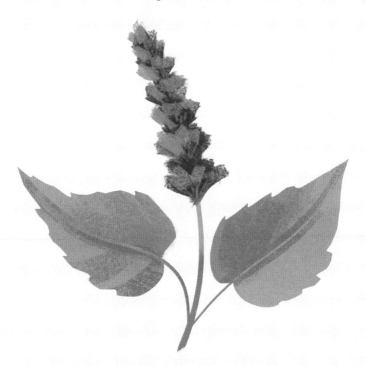

Smell

Earthy
Woody

Essential Facts

Ancient Orient traders would pack their silk bundles with patchouli leaves to keep moths and other bugs away from their valuable cargo!

25

Orrin Oregano

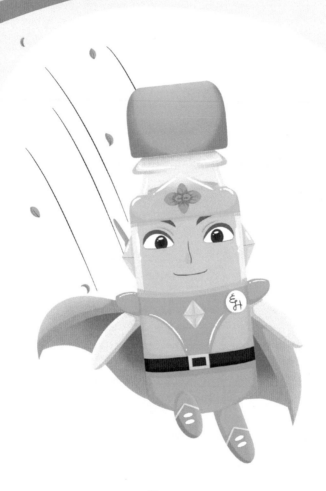

Common Uses for Oregano:
- **Skin Health**
- **Cleansing**
- **Immune Support**

Where in the world?
Oregano oil is distilled from the leaves of plants found in the Mediterranean and Mexico.

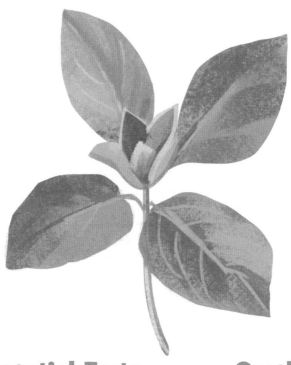

Essential Facts
Oregano is a well known ingredient in pizza, spaghetti, and other tasty Italian dishes!!!

Smell
Sharp

Ollie Orange

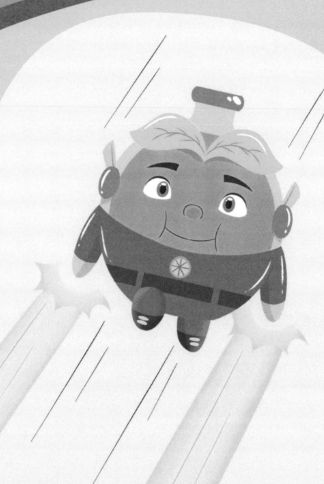

Common Uses for Orange:
- Uplifting
- Cleansing
- Mood Lifter

Where in the world?

Orange oil is cold pressed from the rinds of the orange fruit found in Asia and parts of North America.

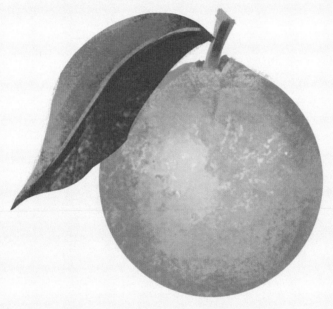

Smell
Sweet
Citrusy
Fresh

Essential Facts
Orange fruit was used for its medicinal properties in ancient China and India before it was widely consumed as a food and drink!!!

Cindy Cinnamon

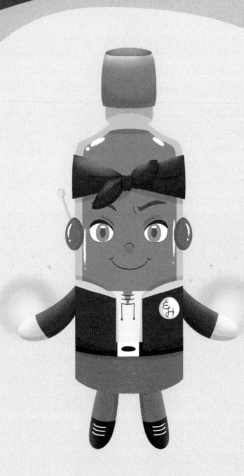

Common Uses for Cinnamon:
- Cleansing
- Immune Support
- Stimulating

Where in the world?

Cinnamon oil is harvested by distilling the bark of cinnamon trees found in India and Madagascar.

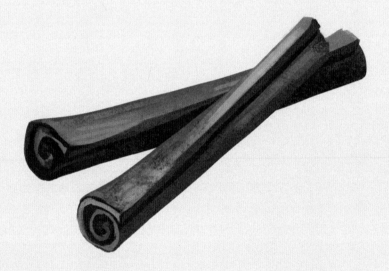

Essential Facts

Before refrigeration and modern food packaging, cinnamon was used for food preservation because of its cleansing and purifying properties

Smell

Spicy
Warm
Sweet

Heidi Helichrysum

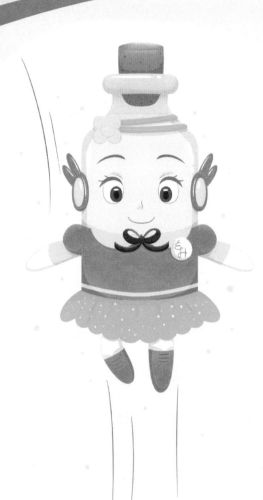

Common Uses for Helichrysum:
- Skin Health
- Cleansing
- Stimulating

Where in the world?

Helichrysum oil is distilled from the flowers
of the plant found in France and Italy.

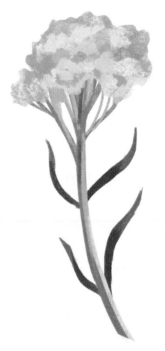

Smell
Rich
Honey
Sweet

Essential Facts
The word helichrysum
literally means "golden spiral"
which describes this plant's
beautiful blossoms!!!

Ned Nutmeg

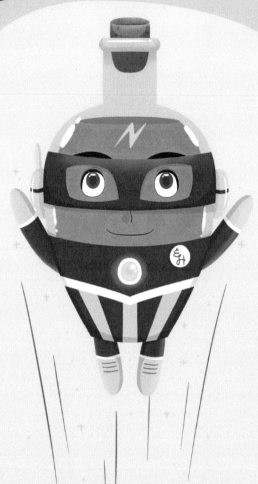

Common Uses for Nutmeg:
- Tummy support
- Cleansing
- Stimulating

Where in the world?

Nutmeg oil is distilled from the fruits and seeds of nutmeg trees found in Indonesia and Tunisia.

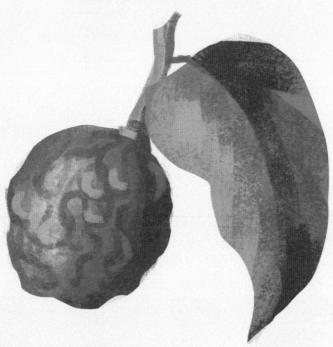

Essential Facts

Afraid of bees? You'd be in good company with nutmeg trees as they are pollinated by beetles, not by bees!!!

Smell

Spicy
Musky
Sweet

Samuel Sandalwood

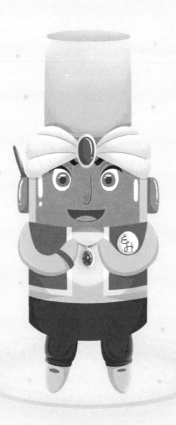

Common Uses for Sandalwood:
- Soothing
- Relaxing
- Cleansing

Where in the world?

Sandalwood oil is distilled from the wood of trees found in India, Indonesia, and Hawaii.

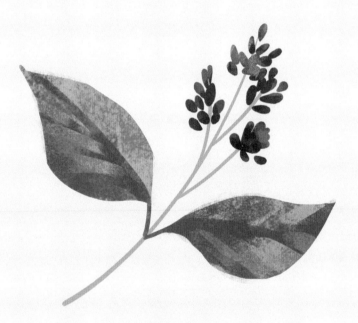

Smell
Soft
Woody
Earthy

Essential Facts
Sandalwood trees need to be at least 30 years old before they can be harvested for essential oil!!!

Yin Yang Ylang Ylang

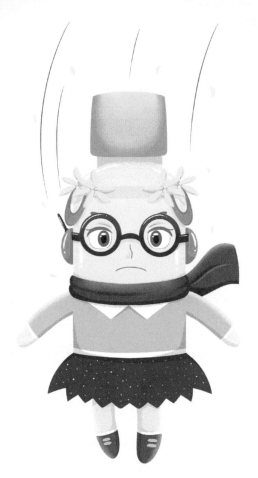

Common Uses for Ylang Ylang:
- **Skin Health**
- **Mood**
- **Balancing**

Where in the world?

Ylang Ylang oil is distilled from blossoms found on trees in Ecuador, the Philippines, and Madagascar.

Essential Facts

The Name Ylang Ylang means "wilderness" which is where these small flowery trees are usually found!!!

Smell

Sweet
Floral

Marjorie Marjoram

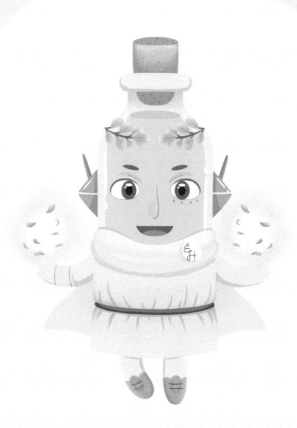

Common Uses for Marjoram:
- Immune Support
- Fatigue
- Soothing

Where in the world?
Marjoram oil is steam distilled from the leaves of plants found in France.

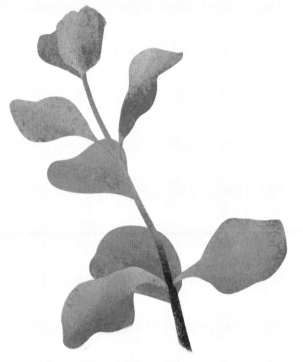

Smell
Spicy

Essential Facts
Marjoram was used in ancient Greek and Roman cultures as a symbol for happiness!!!

Rosa Rosemary

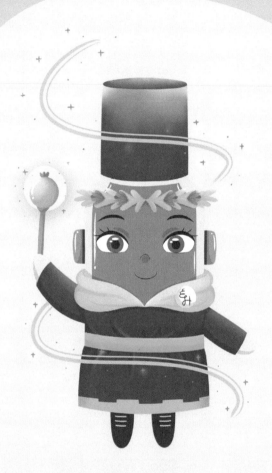

Common Uses for Rosemary:
- Memory Support
- Hair Health
- Mental Clarity

42

Where in the world?

Rosemary oil is distilled from flowering blossoms on evergreen shrubs found in France and North America.

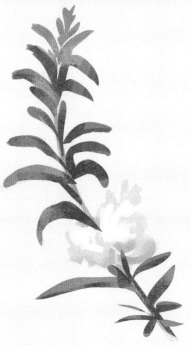

Essential Facts
In the 16th century, Rosemary was used as a household cleaner in Europe!!!

Smell
Woody
Evergreen

Blake Black Spruce

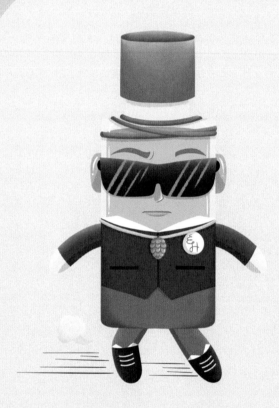

Common Uses for Black Spruce:
- Calming
- Emotional Balance
- Boldness

Where in the world?

Black Spruce oil is distilled from trees found in North America.

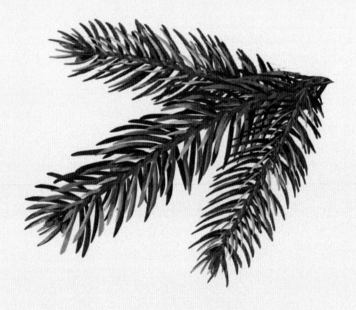

Smell
Fresh
Earthy
Woody

Essential Facts
The Wright Brothers used spruce wood to help build their first airplane called the "Flyer!!!"

Gwendolyn Grapefruit

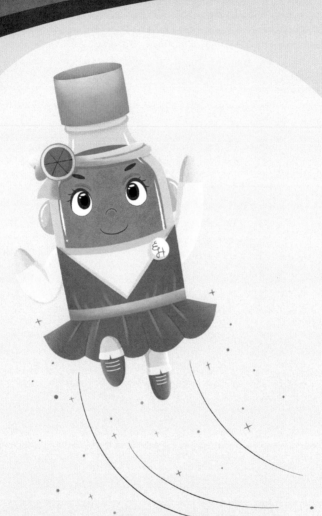

Common Uses for Grapefruit:
- Cleansing
- Skin Healthy
- Uplifting

Where in the world?

Grapefruit oil is cold pressed from the rinds of fruit found in North America and Asia.

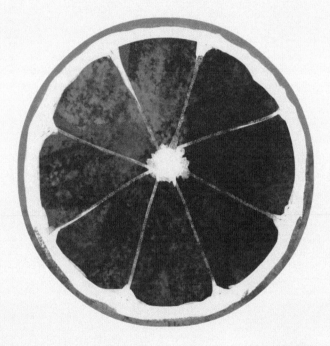

Essential Facts

Grapefruit got its name because the fruit grows in clusters, similar to that of grapes!!!

Smell

Clean
Fresh
Citrusy

Victor Vetiver

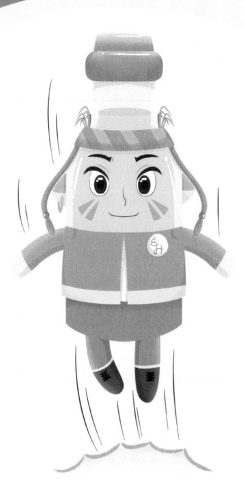

Common Uses for Vetiver:
- Calming
- Emotional Balance
- Boldness

Where in the world?

Vetiver oil is steam distilled from the roots of tall grasses found in India and Haiti.

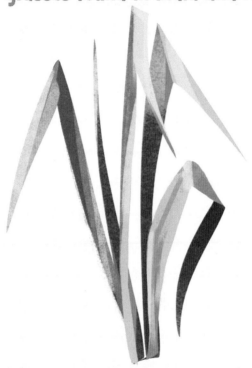

Smell

Earthy
Musky
Smokey

Essential Facts

Vetiver is a long, rigid grass used to build huts in hot parts of the world. The grass holds water long after being cut which helps keep the huts cool!!!

Clarke Clove

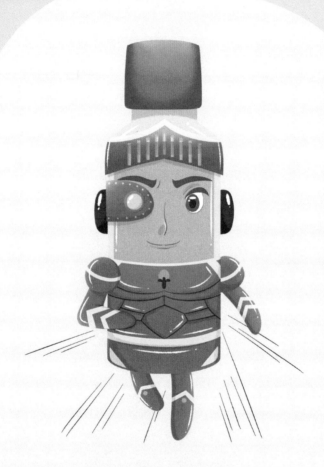

Common Uses for Clove:
- Immune Support
- Cleansing
- Soothing

Where in the world?
Clove oil is distilled from the bud, and stem of plants found in Madagascar, and Indonesia.

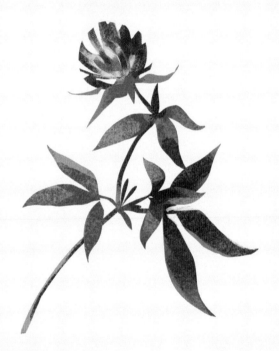

Essential Facts
Clove oil has the highest anti-oxidant property of any other substance on earth!!!

Smell
Spicy
Warm
Woody

Bart Bergamot

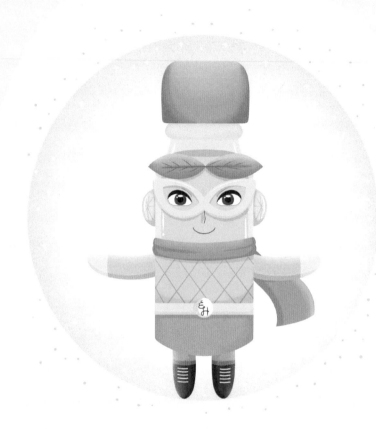

Common Uses for Bergamot:

- Calming
- Uplifting
- Emotional Balance

Where in the world?

Bergamot oil is cold pressed from the rinds of fruits found in Italy and the Ivory Coast.

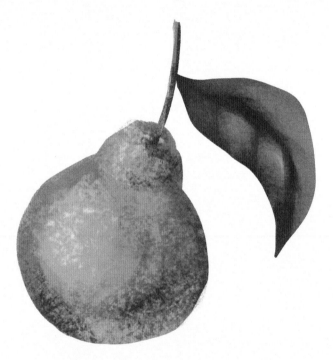

Smell
Sweet
Citrusy
Fruity

Essential Facts
Bergamot is a member of the citrus family which means it is related to oranges, grapefruit, lemons, and limes!!!

Mike Melaleuca

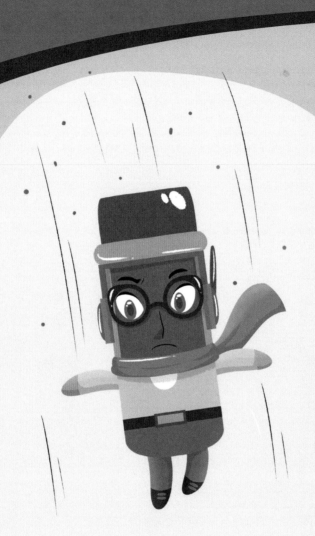

Common Uses for Melaleuca:
- Cleansing
- Odor Control
- Pest Control

54

Where in the world?

Melaleuca oil is steam distilled from the leaves and limbs of plants found in Australia.

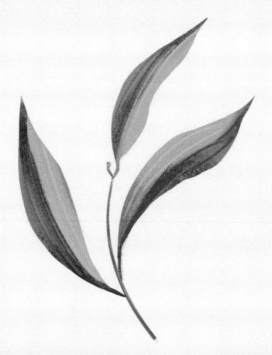

Essential Facts

The melaleuca plant can protect itself from many types of viruses, bacteria, and fungi that infect plants!!!

Smell

Fresh
Earthy
Woody

Lester Lime

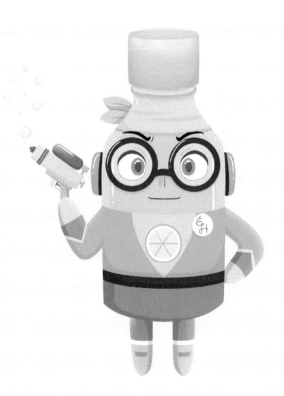

Common Uses for Lime:
- **Uplifting**
- **Emotional Support**
- **Cleansing**

Where in the world?

Bergamot oil is cold pressed from the rinds of fruits found in Italy and the Ivory Coast.

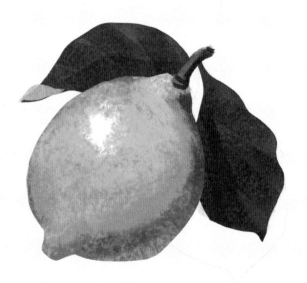

Smell

Sweet
Tart

Essential Facts

Limes have high levels of Vitamin C and were placed aboard old time sailing ships to help sailors avoid a disease called scurvy!!!

Eugene Eucalyptus

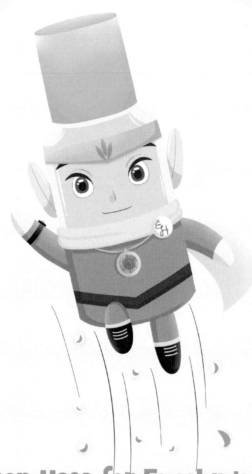

Common Uses for Eucalyptus:
- **Breathing Support**
- **Stimulating**
- **Soothing**

Where in the world?

Eucalyptus oil is steam distilled from the leaves of plants found in Australia, China, and Brazil.

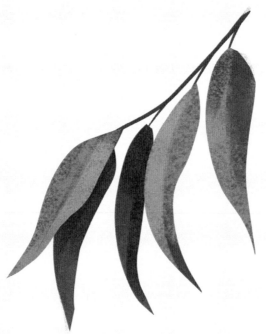

Essential Facts

Eucalyptus family reunions are very big as there are over 700 different types of eucalyptus trees and shrubs in the world!!!

Smell

Woodsy
Fresh
Earthy

Charlotte Chamomile

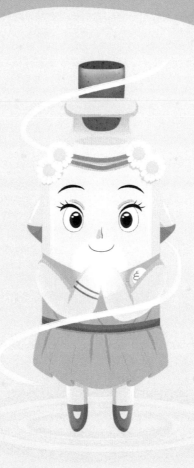

Common Uses for Chamomile:
- Calming
- Emotional Balance
- Skin Health

Where in the world?

Chamomile oil is steam distilled from flowers found in North America and Egypt.

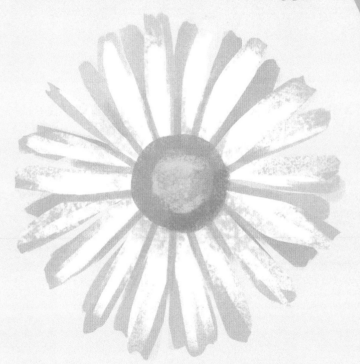

Smell
Fresh
Fruity
Sweet

Essential Facts
The name chamomile means "ground apple." As the name implies, chamomile flowers grow close to the ground and have an apple scent!!!

Safety Tips

1. Never use essential oils without an adult's permission.

2. Do not put essential oils in your eyes or ears.

3. Be careful to avoid sunshine if you have citrus oils (orange, lemon, lime, grapefruit, bergamot) on your skin.

4. NEVER consume essential oils with out an adult's direction.

There is much to learn about essential oils and this guidebook is only the beginning of your journey. Remember to only use essential oils with your parent's permission and always practice oil safety.

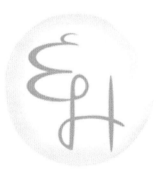

MyEssentialHeroes.Com

Made in the
USA
Lexington, KY